Ketogenic Diet Rapid Weight Loss Holiday Recipes:

Lose Up To 30 LBS. In 30 Days

Henry Brooke

Description

Keto Sourdough Baguettes

Keto Stuffing

Creamy Cauliflower Mashed Potatoes

Keto 'Potato' Salad

Roasted Pecan Green Beans

Keto Creamed Spinach

Keto Au Gratin Brussels Sprouts

Lemon Roasted Spicy Broccoli

Bacon Wrapped Chicken with gravy

Stuffed Pork Tenderloin wrapped with bacon

Bourbon Glazed Ham

Crispy Slow Roasted Pork Shoulder

Oven Roasted Turkey Legs

Sage and Orange glazed Duck Breast

Slow Cooker Braised Oxtails

Stuffed Pork Loin

Slow Cooked Lamb with Green beans and mint

Crock Pot Beef Brisket

Caramel pots de crème

Chocolate, Chia and Orange Pudding

Pumpkin Snickerdoodle Cookies

No Bake Pumpkin Pie Cheesecake

Keto Gingerbread Cake

Keto Peanut Butter Fudge Bars

Keto Hot Cocoa

Introduction

Hanukkah and Christmas dinner may bring fear to those on the ketogenic diet. I bet you are already thinking about how off track you are going to go. But do I have good news for you; there's no need to get off track during the holiday. This cookbook will share with you 30 delicious, holiday-friendly meals that you can enjoy without falling off your diet. This book has recipes that are simple to pull together and that everyone can enjoy even if they aren't on the keto diet. There are meat dishes, side dishes and many desserts that are low in carbs and high in fats so that they are excellent in keeping you in ketosis.

There are many ketogenic books that claim to have low carb recipes but they have starchy items included in their recipes. This cookbook will not disappoint as each recipe makes use of all ingredients that are conducive to maintaining ketosis. The instructions are easy to follow and you don't have to be a professional to create these exceptional dishes. Each meal is followed my nutritional information so you can add up those micronutrients based on your needs. Feel free to make these dishes and share them with all family and friends and they may be asking you for these recipes soon. I certainly hope you enjoy these meals and that they make the holidays happier and easier for you. Enjoy!

Keto Sourdough Baguettes

These low carb baguettes can be freshly made and enjoyed with your holiday meal.

You can even use these to make sandwiches with leftover meats from the holidays.

Serves: 8

Preparation Time: 75 minutes

Ingredients

Dry ingredients:

- Psyllium husk powder (1/3 cup)

- Flax meal (1/2 cup)

- Sea salt (1 teaspoon)

- Almond flour (1 ½ cups)

- Coconut flour (1/2 cup)

- Baking soda (1 ½ teaspoons)

Wet ingredients:

- Eggs (2, large)

- Apple cider vinegar (1/4 cup)

- Egg whites (6, large)

- Buttermilk (3/4 cup, low-fat)

- Water (1 cup, hot)

Directions

1. Set oven to 360°F.

2. Combine dry ingredients together in a bowl.

3. Mix together buttermilk, whites and eggs in a separate bowl.

4. Add mixture to dry mixture and use mixer to combine then add water and vinegar and mix together.

5. Line baking sheet with parchment paper and grease with cooking spray.

6. Spoon mixture onto sheet and shape. Leave spaces between baguettes.

7. Bake for 15 minutes then lower heat to 300°F and bake for 40-45 minutes more.

8. Cool and serve!

Nutritional Facts (per serving)

Calories 232

Fats 16.4g

Protein 12.2g

Net carbs 4.5g

Keto Stuffing

Don't you just wish you could indulge in some stuffing on the holidays? Well try this keto friendly low carb stuffing and stuff your face without regret. Just use the sourdough baguettes to make this treat.

Serves: 8-16

Preparation Time: 4 hours

Ingredients

- Sausage meat (600g, gluten free)

- Onion (1)

- Celery (3 stalks, chopped)

- Rosemary (1 tablespoon, chopped)

- Coconut milk (1/3 cup)

- Salt (1 teaspoon)

- Sourdough baguettes (8)

- Ghee/lard (1/4 cup)

- Garlic (3 cloves)

- Sage (1 tablespoon, fresh, chopped)

- Chicken stock (3 cups)

- Eggs (2)

- Black pepper (1/4 teaspoon)

Directions

1. Slice baguettes into pieces about ½ inch each.

2. Set oven to 210°F.

3. Put bread onto a lined baking sheet and bake for 3 hours until dry. Take from heat and cool.

4. Set oven to 350°F.

5. Take casing from sausage and heat half of ghee in a pot. Add sausage and use spatula to break up meat. Cook for 8 minutes or until meat is golden all over. Remove meat from pot with a slotted spoon and put aside.

6. Chop onion and garlic and add to pot, cook for 10 minutes until slightly golden.

7. Add celery and herbs to pot and cook for 5 minutes or celery is soft.

8. Put sausage, bread and celery mix into a large bowl then add stock and allow bread to soak up liquid.

9. Combine eggs with cream, pepper and salt.

10. Put bread mixture into a baking dish and add egg mixture all over bread.

11.Bake for 40 minutes, remove from heat and serve.

Nutritional Facts (per serving)

Calories 278

Fats 21.7g

Protein 14.3g

Net carbs 3.6g

Creamy Cauliflower Mashed Potatoes

Creamy mashed potatoes are perfect for any holiday meal however potatoes are a no-no on the keto diet. This mashed cauliflower dish will satisfy all those cravings for potatoes, simply delicious!

Serves: 3

Preparation Time: 20 minutes

Ingredients

- Cauliflower (10 oz.)

- Whipping cream (3 tablespoons, heavy)

- Parmesan cheese (4 tablespoons)

- Chives (2 tablespoons, chopped)

- Sour cream (1/4 cup)

- Butter (3 tablespoons)

- Garlic powder (1/4 teaspoon)

- Salt

- Pepper

Directions

1. Put heads of cauliflower a little at a time into a processor and pulse until consistency is similar to rice.

2. Steam cauliflower in a pot for 5 minutes until softened yet firm.

3. Add whipping dream, cheese, sour cream, butter and garlic powder to cauliflower; stir to combine.

4. Use an immersion blender to combine the ingredients together or process in processor again till combined.

5. Top with chives and serve!

Nutritional Facts (per serving)

Calories 251

Fats 21.7g

Protein 6g

Net carbs 4g

Keto 'Potato' Salad

Of course this isn't really a potato salad as all those carbs would throw you out of ketosis. Instead we make use of rutabaga and turnip along other vegetables. With a mayonnaise mustard sauce this salad will be a star at the table.

Serves: 8

Preparation Time: 30 minutes

Ingredients

Spices for cooking vegetables:

- Black peppercorns (1 teaspoon)

- Salt (1/2 teaspoon)

- Apple cider vinegar (1 tablespoon)

- Bay leaves (2)

Dressing and salad:

- Turnip (7.1 oz.)

- Cucumber (4.2 oz., pickled)

- Onion (1)

- Mayonnaise (3/4 cup)

- Vinegar (2 tablespoons)

- Parsley (2 tablespoons)

- Black pepper

- Rutabaga (17.6 oz.)

- Celeriac (5.3 oz.)

- Eggs (6)

- Celery (1 stalk, sliced)

- Dijon mustard (1 teaspoon)

- Celery seeds (1 teaspoon)

- Salt

- Chives (2 tablespoons)

Directions

1. Fill a saucepan with water and add a little salt. Heat water and use a spoon to add eggs to water. Boil for 10 minutes and then remove from hot water and place in cold water.

2. Peel turnip, celeriac and rutabaga and cut into 1" pieces. Rutabaga can be cut smaller than the others as it takes a longer time to cook.

3. Fill a pot with water and add vinegar, salt, bay leaves and peppercorns. Add diced vegetables to pot and bring to a boil. Cook for 15 minutes until rutabaga is cooked.

4. Drain vegetables and remove excess spices. Put aside to cool and then put into a bowl.

5. Dice pickles and onions and add to vegetables. Remove shells from eggs and chop then add to bowl along with vinegar.

6. Put in mustard and mayonnaise, herbs, celery seeds and celery stalk. Mix till thoroughly combined; add pepper and salt to taste.

7. Refrigerate for 2 hours or overnight.

Nutritional Facts (per serving)

Calories 254

Fats 21.1g

Protein 6.6g

Net carbs 7.6g

Roasted Pecan Green Beans

It is best to use dry beans for this recipe so that they can get real crispy. The beans will leave your mouth with a burst of flavor like no other beans you've ever had. The nutty essence will leave you wanting more.

Serves: 4

Preparation Time: 30 minutes

Ingredients

- Olive oil (1/4 cup)
- Parmesan cheese (1/4 cup)
- Garlic (2 teaspoons, diced)
- Green beans (1 lb.)
- Pecans (1/2 cup, chopped)
- Lemon zest (from 1 lemon)
- Red pepper flakes (1 teaspoon)

Directions

1. Set oven to 450°F.

2. Put pecans in processor and grind till chopped coarsely.

3. Add pecans to a bowl along with all remaining ingredients.

4. Line a baking sheet with foil and spread mixture onto foil.

5. Roast for 25 minutes, turning to avoid burning if necessary.

6. Cool for 5 minutes and serve!

Nutritional Facts (per serving)

Calories 273

Fats 25.3g

Protein 5.5g

Net carbs 5g

Keto Creamed Spinach

This bright green vegetable is quick and simple to prepare and everyone may actually give spinach a chance with this creamy side.

Serves: 3

Preparation Time: 15 minutes

Ingredients

- Spinach (10 oz.)

- Cream cheese (3 tablespoons)

- Garlic powder (1/4 teaspoon)

- Salt

- Parmesan cheese (3 tablespoons)

- Sour cream (2 tablespoons)

- Onion powder

- Pepper

- Olive oil

Directions

1. Rinse spinach and drain.

2. Heat a deep skillet and use a little oil to grease pot. Add spinach to pot and cook for about 5 minutes until wilted.

3. Add garlic and onion powder along with cream cheese to spinach and stir to combine. Cook until cheese melts.

4. Add parmesan and sour cream, stir to combine and cook until mixture is thick; add pepper and salt to taste.

5. Serve!

Nutritional Facts (per serving)

Calories 157

Fats 13.3g

Protein 5.7g

Net carbs 2g

Keto Au Gratin Brussels Sprouts

Who says you have to prepare your sprouts the same old way all the time. For the holidays dress up your sprouts in a cheesy au gratin and impress all who indulge in this delight.

Serves: 4

Preparation Time: 40 minutes

Ingredients

- Brussels sprouts (6 oz.)
- Garlic (1 teaspoon, diced)
- Soy sauce (1 tablespoon)
- Pepper (1/4 teaspoon)
- Onion (1.8 oz.)
- Butter (2 tablespoon)
- Liquid smoke (1/2 teaspoon)

For cheese sauce:

- Heavy cream (1/2 cup)

- Paprika (1/4 teaspoon)

- Pepper (1/4 teaspoon)

- Butter (1 tablespoon)

- Cheddar cheese (2.5 oz., shredded)

- Turmeric (1/4 teaspoon)

- Xanthan gum (1/8 teaspoon)

For crust:

- Parmesan cheese (3 tablespoons)

- Pork rinds (0.5 oz.)

- Paprika (1/2 teaspoon)

Directions

1. Set oven to 375°F.

2. Cut stems from sprouts and slice in halves. Dice garlic and chop onion.

3. Melt butter in a skillet and add sprouts; cook for 3 minutes then add garlic, onion and pepper. Cook for 3 minutes until onion gets soft.

4. Add liquid smoke and soy sauce and remove from heat.

5. Put all ingredients for cheese sauce in a saucepan and heat thoroughly until sauce thickens. Stir to avoid burning.

6. Add sprouts to sauce and combine then spoon into ramekins.

7. Put ingredients for crust in a grinder and grind together. Use mixture to top sprouts.

8. Bake for 20 minutes until crust is slightly crisp.

9. Serve!

Nutritional Facts (per serving)

Calories 303

Fats 27.3g

Protein 9.5g

Net carbs 4.5g

Lemon Roasted Spicy Broccoli

Broccoli is one of those things that can usually seem bland or boring. Try this lemon spicy mixture for the holidays and even the kids won't be able to resist.

Serves: 6

Preparation Time: 25 minutes

Ingredients

- Parmesan cheese (1/3 cup)

- Basil (2 tablespoons, chopped)

- Kosher salt (1/2 teaspoon)

- Lemon zest (from ½ lemon)

- Broccoli florets (1 ½ lbs.)

- Olive oil (1/4 cup)

- Garlic (3 teaspoons, diced)

- Red chili flakes (1/2 teaspoon)

- Lime juice (from ½ lemon)

Directions

1. Set oven to 425°F.

2. Put broccoli in a Ziploc bag along with all ingredients except cheese. Shake to combine.

3. Line a baking sheet with parchment paper and put broccoli onto sheet. Top with cheese.

4. Bake for 20 minutes, turning if necessary.

5. Take from oven and serve!

Nutritional Facts (per serving)

Calories 137

Fats 10.5g

Protein 5.7g

Net carbs 3.7g

Bacon Wrapped Chicken with gravy

This is a great way to prepare your chicken for the holidays. Anything wrapped in bacon is most definitely always a treat. Can be paired with the Keto Au Gratin sprouts and you will truly enjoy every bite.

Serves: 8

Preparation Time: 1 hour 20 minutes

Ingredients

- Whole chicken (3lbs., gutted)
- Lemon (1, sliced)
- Bacon (10 strips)
- Salt
- Thyme (4 sprigs, fresh)
- Lime (1, sliced)
- Grain mustard (1 tablespoon)
- Pepper

Directions

1. Set oven to 500°F. Use pepper and salt to season the chicken and then stuff with lemon, thyme and lime.

2. Use bacon to wrap chicken; overlapping if necessary (you may use more bacon if necessary). Sprinkle with pepper and salt.

3. Place chicken into a roasting pan and roast for 15 minutes then lower heat to 350°F. Bake for 40-50 minutes more.

4. Take chicken from oven and wrap in foil and put aside.

5. Pour liquid from roasting pan into a saucepan and add mustard. Stir to combine and use a whisk to blend (you may use your immersion blender if you have one). Cook until slightly thick.

6. Serve gravy with chicken.

Nutritional Facts (per serving)

Calories 376

Fats 29.8g

Protein 24.5g

Net carbs 1.5g

Stuffed Pork Tenderloin wrapped with bacon

Christmas time is usually the time a year where pork rules most households. If you aren't interested in doing the traditional ham, how about this easy to make tenderloin that will make you look like you took extra effort to prepare. You can prepare the tenderloin alone or with the vegetable sauté in this recipe.

Serves: 4

Preparation Time: 1 hour 25 minutes

Ingredients

- Pork tenderloin (16 oz.)
- Onion (1/2, chopped)
- Olive oil (1 tablespoon)
- Cream cheese (3 oz.)
- Thyme (1/2 teaspoon, dried)
- Salt
- Bacon (14 slices)
- Garlic (2 teaspoons, diced)
- Spinach (2 oz.)

- Liquid smoke (1/2 teaspoon, optional)

- Rosemary (1/2 teaspoon)

- Pepper

For Vegetable Sauté:

- Broccoli (4 oz., chopped)

- Tomatoes (1/2 cup, diced)

- Garlic powder (1/2 teaspoon)

- Bell pepper (1/2, orange)

- Onion powder (1/2 teaspoon)

- Pepper

Directions

1. Heat oil in a skillet and sauté onion for 3 minutes until it gets soft.

2. Add garlic, stir and cook for 1 minute then put in spinach. Add spices except, ¼ teaspoon rosemary, ¼ teaspoon thyme and ¼ teaspoon liquid smoke. Cook spinach till wilted then add cheese. Remove from heat and put aside.

3. Set oven to 350°F.

4. Put tenderloin on a flat surface (preferably a cutting board). Use a meat hammer to pound meat until it is flat then slice edges to form a square. Use pepper and salt to season meat.

5. Arrange bacon slices in a woven design on a flat surface (similar to a basket), should be the same size as the tenderloin.

6. Place tenderloin on top of bacon and top with spinach and add cream cheese.

7. Roll tenderloin into a log and use toothpicks to hold ends together.

8. Bake for 75 minutes and use thermometer to check meat. If it reads 140°F then meat is ready. Turn off over oven and let meat sit.

9. Use drippings from pork to sauté vegetables.

10. Serve!

Nutritional Facts (per serving)

Tenderloin only

Calories 606

Fats 51.8g

Protein 30g

Net carbs 2.8g

Tenderloin and vegetables

Nutritional Facts (per serving)

Calories 627

Fats 51.8g

Protein 31.3g

Net carbs 6g

Bourbon Glazed Ham

Standing tall on many holiday tables is the beloved ham. This bourbon glazed ham could be a great twist on your ham this year. The simple ingredients work together to make a bold impression.

Serves: 12

Preparation Time: 2 hours 15 minutes

Ingredients

- Ham shank (8-12 lbs., bone in)
- Mustard (1 teaspoon, ground)
- Bourbon (2 oz.)
- Splenda (1 ¼ cup)
- Champagne vinegar (1 teaspoon)
- Cloves

Directions

1. Set oven to 325°F.

2. Remove excess fat from ham and use knife to score ham in a crisscross pattern.

3. Put into a roasting pan with about 2 inches of water and cook in over, covered for 1 hour.

4. Combine all remaining ingredients in a saucepan except cloves. Heat mixture until it comes to a boil.

5. Take ham from oven and drain water reserving a little in pan.

6. Push cloves into opening on ham and glaze ham.

7. Return to over without cover and cook for 1 hour. Add more glaze if necessary.

8. Remove from heat, cool, slice and serve!

Nutritional Facts (per serving)

Calories 548

Fats 32g

Protein 50g

Net carbs 6g

Crispy Slow Roasted Pork Shoulder

If you like roasts on your table for the holiday then try this succulent pork roast with a crispy outer. This is a meal that can feed a crowd and if you are looking for something that is not too expensive this is your best bet. It does take a while to make but it will be worth it.

Serves: 20

Preparation Time: 11 hours

Ingredients

- Pork shoulder (8 lbs.)
- Oregano (2 teaspoons)
- Garlic powder (1 teaspoon)
- Salt (3 ½ tablespoons)
- Black pepper (1 teaspoon)
- Onion powder (1 teaspoon)

Directions

1. Rinse pork and pat dry then allow it to sit until it gets to room temperature.

2. Set oven to 250°F and combine all remaining ingredients in a bowl.

3. Rub dry mixture all over pork.

4. Line baking sheet with foil and place a rack on top of it. Place pork onto rack and bake for 8-10 hours.

5. Take from oven and put aside covered; put aside for 15 minutes.

6. Set oven to 500°F.

7. Take foil from pork and roast for an additional 20 minutes, turning every 5 minutes.

8. Remove from heat and sit for 20 minutes.

9. Slice and serve!

Nutritional Facts (per serving)

Calories 461

Fats 36.7g

Protein 30.3g

Net carbs 0.2g

Oven Roasted Turkey Legs

If you love turkey but don't want to have to prepare a whole bird; try these turkey legs instead. They are full of flavor and are relatively easy to make.

Serves: 4

Preparation Time: 1 hour

Ingredients

- Turkey legs (2, medium-about a lb. each)

- Salt (2 teaspoons)

- Cayenne pepper (1/4 teaspoon)

- Garlic powder (1/2 teaspoon)

- Ancho chili powder (1/2 teaspoon)

- Worcestershire sauce (1 teaspoon)

- Duck fat/animal fat/peanut oil (2 tablespoons)

- Pepper (1/2 teaspoon)

- Onion powder (1/2 teaspoon)

- Thyme (1/2 teaspoon, dried)

- Liquid smoke (1 teaspoon)

Directions

1. Combine all dry ingredients in a bowl then add liquids and stir together.

2. Rinse turkey legs and pat dry then use mixture to rub all over turkey legs.

3. Set oven to 350°F.

4. Heat fat in a cast iron until it starts to smoke then put in turkey and sear on each side for 2 minutes.

5. Take cast iron from stove and put into oven. Bake for 50 minutes or until cooked thoroughly.

6. Serve!

Nutritional Facts (per serving)

Calories 382

Fats 22.5g

Protein 44g

Net carbs 0.8g

Sage and Orange glazed Duck Breast

If you are planning something really fancy then this glazed duck is sure to make a lasting impression. The sauce is incredible and you could easily try cooking other meats such as chicken with it.

Serves: 1

Preparation Time:

Ingredients

- Duck breast (6 oz.)

- Heavy cream (1 tablespoon)

- Orange extract (1/2 teaspoon)

- Spinach (1 cup)

- Butter (2 tablespoons)

- Splenda sweetener (1 tablespoon)

- Sage (1/2 teaspoon)

Directions

1. Use knife to score skin on top of duck breast and use pepper and salt to season.

2. Put sweetener and butter in a pan and heat till mixture is slightly golden.

3. Add extract and sage and stir to combine; cook until mixture has an amber color.

4. Place duck into a cold pan and place over a medium flame. Cook until crisp on one side then flip.

5. Add cream to butter mixture and combine. Add mixture to duck and cook for about 5 minutes.

6. Add spinach to pot that sauce was made in. Cook until spinach is wilted.

7. Serve spinach with duck breast and sauce.

Nutritional Facts (per serving)

Calories 798

Fats 71g

Protein 36g

Net carbs 0g

Slow Cooker Braised Oxtails

Oxtail meat can be an enjoyable experience if cooked right. This meat is a delicacy in many places and for good reason. The meat just gets so soft after being cooked and are great with cauliflower mashed 'potatoes'.

Serves: 3

Preparation Time:

Ingredients

- Oxtail (2 lbs.)
- Soy sauce (2 tablespoons)
- Tomato paste (3 tablespoons)
- Garlic (1 teaspoon, diced)
- Butter (1/3 cup)
- Salt
- Beef broth (2 cups)
- Fish sauce (1 tablespoon)
- Onion powder (1 teaspoon)
- Ginger (1/2 teaspoon, ground)

- Thyme (1 teaspoon, dried)

- Guar gum (1/2 teaspoon, optional)

- **Pepper**

Directions

1. Put broth into a saucepan and bring to a boil then add soy sauce, tomato paste, butter and fish sauce.

2. Season oxtail with spices and put into slow cooker and add sauce to cooker.

3. Cook for 6-7 hours on low setting.

4. Take oxtails from gravy and put aside. Add gum to gravy and whisk to combine until thick.

5. Serve oxtail with gravy and your favorite side.

Nutritional Facts (per serving)

Calories 433

Fats 29.7g

Protein 28.3g

Net carbs 3.2g

Stuffed Pork Loin

Do you love pumpkins? You can incorporate pumpkins in this tender pork loin and this fatty succulent pork will be in your memories long after you've enjoyed it.

Serves: 8

Preparation Time: 1 hour 30 minutes

Ingredients

- Pork loin (3 lbs.)
- Ghee (2 tablespoons)
- Garlic (4 cloves, diced)
- Chorizo sausage (3/5 oz., chopped)
- Salt (1 teaspoon)
- Sausage meat (1 lb., gluten free)
- Onion (1, chopped)
- Pumpkin (2 cups, diced)
- Rosemary (1 tablespoon, chopped)
- Black pepper (1/2 teaspoon)
- Sage (1 tablespoon, chopped)

Directions

1. Set oven to 450°F. Take casing from sausage and heat a tablespoon of ghee in a pot.

2. Cook sausage for 8 minutes until golden using spatula to break up meat. Take meat from pot with a slotted spoon and put into a large bowl.

3. Add leftover ghee to pot along with onion and garlic. Cook for 10 minutes until golden then add rosemary, sage and chorizo; cook for 2 minutes.

4. Add pumpkin and cook for 10 minutes, take from heat and add to sausage in bowl and combine.

5. Use a knife to score skin of loin.

6. Use a sharp knife to slice loin lengthwise so that you have a flat loin that can be rolled up.

7. If meat is thick, use a mallet to pound flat. Add stuffing leaving about an inch from all edges. Roll loin trying to roll as tight as possible. Tie meat in place or use a netting to hold in place. Use pepper and salt to season.

8. Place into a baking dish and bake for 20 minutes then lower heat to 325°F and cook for an additional 40 minutes or until thoroughly cooked.

9. Remove from heat, cover and let meat sit at least 10 minutes before slicing.

Nutritional Facts (per serving)

Calories 540

Fats 36.4g

Protein 46.5g

Net carbs 3.9g

Slow Cooked Lamb with Green beans and mint

Slow cooking meats gives your meat lots of flavor while cooking and is great way to prepare healthy meals without having to stand over a hot stove all day. You can prepare this meal aside while you finish up your other holiday foods.

Serves: 4

Preparation Time: 6-10 hours

Ingredients

- Lamb leg (3lbs with bone)
- Garlic (4 cloves, chopped)
- Green beans (6 cups, trimmed)
- Black pepper
- Ghee (2 tablespoons)
- Mint (1/4 cup, fresh, chopped)
- Salt (1/2 teaspoon)

Directions

1. Turn on slow cooker and dry lamb with paper towel. Use pepper and salt to season lamb.

2. Heat a large pot and melt ghee then add lamb to pot and fry on both sides until golden.

3. Put lamb into slow cooker along with mint and garlic. Add water if necessary and set on low for 10 hours or high for 6 hours.

4. Before final 2 hours of cooking, remove meat and put beans into cooker then top with lamb. Cook for remaining time.

5. Let meat sit a little after cooking, slice and serve with beans.

Nutritional Facts (per serving)

Calories 524

Fats 36.4g

Protein 37.3g

Net carbs 7.6g

Crock Pot Beef Brisket

Brisket is perfect for slow cooking as the meat is tough so it can be cooked in a lot of liquids. Slow cooking ensures that the meat is slowly infused with all the spices added to the pot. This is a dish that you can enjoy whether you celebrate Christmas or Hanukkah.

Serves: 12

Preparation Time: 7 hours

Ingredients

- Brisket (5 lbs.)
- Water (3/4 cup)
- Bay leaves (4)
- Garlic (3 cloves)
- Pepper (1/4 teaspoon)
- Tomato sauce (1/2 cup)
- Vinegar (1 teaspoon)
- Thyme (1/2 teaspoon)
- Salt (1 teaspoon)

Directions

1. Place brisket into slow cooker.

2. Combine leftover ingredients and pour over meat.

3. Set slow cooker to low and cook for 6-7 hours. Add water as needed.

4. Serve with desired side.

Nutritional Facts (per serving)

Calories 595

Fats 50g

Protein 32g

Net carbs 1g

Caramel pots de crème

You could make these small or large if you prefer. Pots de crème leave a lot of room to be creative as you can make them taste anyway with various extracts.

Serves: 4

Preparation Time: minutes

Ingredients

- Heavy cream (1 ½ cups)

- Liquid stevia (1/4 teaspoon)

- Egg yolks (4, large)

- Maple syrup (1 tablespoon)

- Maple extract (1 teaspoon)

- NOW Erythritol (1/4 cup, powder)

- Salt (1/4 teaspoon)

- Water (6 tablespoons)

- Vanilla extract (1/2 teaspoon)

Directions

1. Set oven to 300°F.

2. Separate whites from yolks and put whites away for use later on. Grind erythritol and put into a saucepan with water. Cook until mixture starts to boil.

3. Combine stevia, vanilla, maple extract, cream and salt in another saucepan. Cook until mixture starts boiling then lower heat and mix.

4. Add maple syrup to erythritol and combine and cook until a runny syrup is formed.

5. Add erythritol mix slowly to cream blend and whisk together. Add a little of the mixture at a time to the eggs and mix to thoroughly combined.

6. Pour into ramekins. Add water to a deep baking sheet and place ramekins on top; bake for 40 minutes.

7. Cool and serve!

Nutritional Facts (per serving)

Calories 359

Fats 34.9g

Protein 2.8g

Net carbs 3g

Chocolate, Chia and Orange Pudding

Making a pudding is a simple way to get creative with a dessert that is not overpowering after a heavy holiday dinner.

Serves: 1

Preparation Time: 15 minutes

Ingredients

- Chia seeds (1/4 cup)

- Almond milk (1/2 cup)

- Erythritol (1 tablespoon, powdered)

- Dark chocolate (2 tablespoons, 85%)

- Coconut milk (1/4 cup)

- Orange zest (1/2 teaspoon)

- Stevia extract (5-10 drops, orange)

- Whipped cream (for topping)

Directions

1. Combine coconut milk, almond milk, erythritol and chia seeds in a bowl.

   You may blend if you prefer a smoother texture.

2. Add zest to mixture along with Stevia.

3. Refrigerate for 15 minutes or overnight if possible.

4. Stir in chocolate before serving and top with whipped cream.

Nutritional Facts (per serving)

Calories 357

Fats 29.2g

Protein 9.2g

Net carbs 6.9g

Pumpkin Snickerdoodle Cookies

Grab one of these during the winter season with a cup of tea and feel relaxed. These snickerdoodles are certainly comfort food.

Serves: 15

Preparation Time: 25 minutes

Ingredients

Cookies:

- Butter (1/4 cup, salted)

- Vanilla extract (1 teaspoon)

- Egg (1)

- Liquid stevia (25 drops)

- Almond flour (1 ½ cups)

- Pumpkin puree (1/2 cup)

- Baking powder (1/2 teaspoon)

- Erythritol (1/4 cup)

For topping:

- Erythritol (2 teaspoons)

- Pumpkin pie spice (1 teaspoon)

Directions

1. Set oven to 350°F.

2. Combine dry ingredients together in a bowl.

3. Put butter, vanilla, stevia and puree in another bowl microwave to heat and whisk together.

4. Add mixture dry ingredients along with egg and combine forming dough.

5. Roll into 15 balls and place on a lined baking sheet and flatten with hand. Bake for 13 minutes covered with foil.

6. Grind topping ingredients in a grinder. Top cookies with mixture as soon as they are finished.

7. Cool and serve!

Nutritional Facts (per serving)

Calories 99

Fats 8.9g

Protein 2.9g

Net carbs 1.7g

No Bake Pumpkin Pie Cheesecake

Who doesn't love cheesecake? Make these to impress your friends and family and they will be in smooth pumpkin cheesecake heaven.

Serves: 8

Preparation Time: 4 hours 15 minutes

Ingredients

For crust:

- Almond flour (3/4 cup)

- Butter (1/4 cup)

- Liquid Stevia (25 drops)

- Flaxseed meal (1/2 cup)

- Pumpkin pie spice (1 teaspoon)

For filling:

- Cream cheese (4 oz.)

- Sour cream (2 tablespoons)

- Butter (3 tablespoons)

- Liquid stevia (25 drops)

- Pumpkin puree (1/3 cup)

- Heavy cream (1/4 cup)

- Pumpkin pie spice (1/4 teaspoon)

Directions

1. Combine all dry ingredients for making crust. Add stevia and butter and mix to combine.

2. Roll into 8 balls and press into individual tart pans.

3. Put all ingredients for filling in a processor and pulse till smooth.

4. Spoon onto crusts and smooth. Chill for at least 4 hours.

5. Top with whipped cream if so desired and serve!

Nutritional Facts (per serving)

Calories 265

Fats 25.3g

Protein 5g

Net carbs 3g

Keto Gingerbread Cake

The smell of this gingerbread cake will have you wanting a slice as soon as it comes out the oven. It is super moist and can be topped with whipped cream and served as a dessert.

Serves: 10

Preparation Time: 1 hour 10 minutes

Ingredients

- Almond flour (2 ¼ cups)

- Coconut flour (2 tablespoons)

- Ginger (1 ½ tablespoons, ground)

- Baking powder (2 teaspoons)

- Salt (1/4 teaspoon)

- Eggs (4)

- Vanilla extract (1 teaspoon)

- Erythritol sweetener (3/4 cup)

- Cocoa powder (1 tablespoon)

- Cinnamon (1/2 tablespoon)

- Ground cloves (1/2 teaspoon)

- Ghee (1/2 cup)

- Almond milk (2/3 cup, unsweetened)

Directions

1. Set oven to 360°F.

2. Put all dry ingredients in a large bowl.

3. Combine all wet ingredients in another bowl and add to dry ingredients; mix together until combined.

4. Spread the mixture in a silicone loaf pan.

5. Bake for 50 minutes until thoroughly baked.

6. Serve!

Nutritional Facts (per serving)

Calories 275

Fats 23g

Protein 9g

Net carbs 7.5g

Keto Peanut Butter Fudge Bars

These bars are easy to love after all when has a peanut butter and chocolate combination ever failed? The bitter taste of the dark chocolate is balanced by the sweet peanut butter fudge and it is something the kids will love too.

Serves: 8

Preparation Time: 10 minutes (plus chilling time)

Ingredients

For crust:

- Butter (1/4 cup, melted)
- Cinnamon (1/2 teaspoon)
- Salt
- Almond flour (1 cup)
- Erythritol (1 tablespoon)

For fudge:

- Heavy cream (1/4 cup)

- Peanut butter (1/2 cup)

- Vanilla extract (1/2 teaspoon)

- Butter (1/4 cup, melted)

- Erythritol (1/4 cup)

- Xanthan gum (1/8 teaspoon)

Topping:

- Chocolate (1/3 cup, chopped)

Directions

1. Set oven to 400°F.

2. Combine all ingredients for crust in a bowl.

3. Line a baking dish with parchment paper, grease with cooking spray and press crust into dish. Bake for 10 minutes and remove from heat.

4. Put ingredients for fudge into a processor and pulse until smooth. Spread fudge all over crust evenly.

5. Top with chocolate and chill overnight.

6. Slice and serve!

Nutritional Facts (per serving)

Calories 300

Fats 19.8g

Protein 4g

Net carbs 3.3g

Keto Hot Cocoa

Nothing says the holidays like a cup of hot cocoa. Pair these with a slice of gingerbread cake of cookies and curl up with your family for a most relaxing time.

Serves: 2

Preparation Time:

Ingredients

- Coconut milk (1 ½ cups, unsweetened)

- Cocoa powder (2 tablespoons, unsweetened)

- Vanilla extract (2 teaspoons)

- Splenda (1 tablespoon)

- Heavy cream (2 tablespoons)

- Instant coffee (1 teaspoon)

- Cinnamon (1/2 teaspoon)

Directions

1. Put cream and coconut milk in a saucepan and heat over a medium flame.

2. As the mixture heats add coffee, cinnamon and cocoa.

3. Add Splenda and vanilla and stir until smooth then bring to a boil and lower flame.

4. Remove from flame; let it sit for 2 minutes then serve!

Nutritional Facts (per serving)

Calories 103

Fats 9g

Protein 1g

Net carbs 3g

Keto Eggnog

This eggnog is a treat for the adults who love to indulge a little alcohol. This creamy nog will certainly put you in the holiday mood.

Serves: 5

Preparation Time: 30 minutes

Ingredients

- Heavy cream (2 cups)
- Eggs (4, large)
- Rum
- Cinnamon (2 teaspoons)
- Coconut milk (1 cup)
- Splenda (4 tablespoons)
- Vanilla (1 tablespoon)
- Allspice (1 teaspoon)

Directions

1. Put milk and cream in a mixing bowl.

2. Separate 3 yolks from whites in to container. Beat egg whites till peaks form and whisk yolks.

3. Add yolks to cream mixture and whisk to combine then add whites and whisk.

4. Add vanilla and spices and continue whisking until mixture is smooth. Beat the leftover egg and add to eggnog.

5. Add desired amount of rum and stir.

6. Refrigerate overnight and serve!

Nutritional Facts (per serving)

Calories 507

Fats 37g

Protein 4.8g

Net carbs 2.9g

Brown Butter Pecan Ice Cream

If you are craving a slice of pecan pie this holiday but you just can't find a recipe to satisfy that sweet tooth. How about a pecan ice cream? The sweet and salty taste is great and will definitely satisfy that craving for pecan pie.

Serves: 4

Preparation Time: 10 minutes (plus freezing time)

Ingredients

- Coconut milk (1 ½ cups, unsweetened)
- Butter (5 tablespoons)
- Liquid stevia (25 drops)
- Heavy cream (1/4 cup)
- Pecans (1/4 cup, crushed)
- Xanthan gum (1/4 teaspoon)

Directions

1. Heat a pot and melt butter. Cook until butter is slightly brown.

2. Add stevia, pecans and cream and mix together.

3. Add gum and coconut milk and whisk into mixture then put into an ice cream maker. Process according to instructions.

4. Top with additional crushed pecans and serve!

Nutritional Facts (per serving)

Calories 319

Fats 35.5g

Protein 0.7g

Net carbs 1.3g

Coffee Ice Cream

So maybe you don't have an ice cream machine at home and that's no reason not to make ice cream at all. How about trying this coffee ice cream? No need for churning.

Serves: 8

Preparation Time: 1 hour 20 minutes (plus freezing time)

Ingredients

- Heavy cream (2 ½ cups)

- Swerve sweetener (1/2 cup, powdered)

- Xanthan gum (1/4 teaspoon)

- Vanilla extract (1/4 teaspoon)

- Almond milk (1 cup, unsweetened)

- Butter (1 tablespoon)

- Instant coffee (1 ½ tablespoons)

- Liquid stevia (1/4 teaspoon)

Directions

1. Pour almond milk and 1 cup of cream into a saucepan. Heat over a medium flame and bring to a boil then lower heat. Slowly cook for about 60 minutes until reduced by half.

2. Take from flame and add butter and sweetener, whisk to combine and add gum.

3. Mix together and add stevia, vanilla and coffee. Whisk some more until mixture is smooth.

4. Whip leftover cream until peaks form then add to milk mixture and fold until combined thoroughly.

5. Put into a freezer safe container and freeze for at least 6 hours or overnight.

6. Serve!

Nutritional Facts (per serving)

Calories 285

Fats 27.8g

Protein 1.7g

Net carbs 2.3g

Jicama Latkes

These treats are a Jewish treat that are usually made around Hanukkah. Many treats are sweet or very fatty and can be excellent for the keto dieter. Latkes are like fritters and they are very simple to whip up.

Serves: 12

Preparation Time: 15 minutes

Ingredients

- Jicama (1 lb.)
- Egg (1, beaten)
- Olive oil (1/2 cup)
- Onion (1/2 cup, diced)
- Salt (1/2 teaspoon)

Directions

1. Use a grater to shred jicama and place onto a clean cloth. Squeeze to remove excess water.
2. Put into a bowl with salt, onion and egg. Stir to combine.

3. Heat oil in a skillet and spoon mixture into pot. Fry for 3-5 minutes on both sides.

4. Place on paper towels to remove excess oil.

5. Serve.

Nutritional Facts (per serving)

Calories 139

Fats 14g

Protein 1g

Net carbs 1g

Zucchini Latkes

Jicama may be a bit hard to acquire for some person so how about trying this zucchini version. It is equally as good as the original.

Serves: 12

Preparation Time: 15 minutes

Ingredients

- Zucchini (1 lb.)

- Egg (1, beaten)

- Olive oil (1/2 cup)

- Onion (1/2 cup, diced)

- Salt (1/2 teaspoon)

Directions

1. Use a grater to shred zucchini and place onto a clean cloth. Squeeze to remove excess water.

2. Put into a bowl with salt, onion and egg. Stir to combine.

3. Heat oil in a skillet and spoon mixture into pot. Fry for 3-5 minutes on both sides.

4. Place on paper towels to remove excess oil.

5. Serve.

Nutritional Facts (per serving)

Calories 131

Fats 14g

Protein 1g

Net carbs 1g